EASY HEALTHCARE:

HEALTHCARE PRIVACY

By

Lori-Ann Rickard

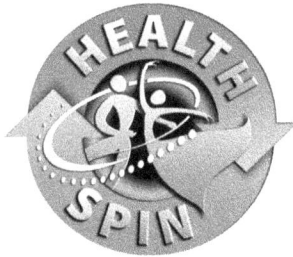

Presented by
Expert Health Press

ISBN-10: 1940767083

ISBN-13: 978-1-940767-08-6

For Alyssa and Cassie, to our next chapter....

TABLE OF CONTENTS

INTRODUCTION

Healthcare has changed radically. Gone are the days when the only medical professional a patient saw was the trusted local doctor. Healthcare is now a massive industry involving any number of people and facilities. Patients and doctors now regularly interact with a long list of groups, including laboratories, imagining companies, hospitals, physical therapists, rehabilitation facilities, nursing homes, assisted living facilities, and insurance companies, to name just a few.

In this complex web of care, your medical records and other sensitive information are seen by dozens of people and live in any number of paper or electronic files stored in an office, on laptops, and thumb drives. They also repeatedly change hands. Therefore, it is important to understand what your privacy rights are and insist that your healthcare information is being protected as much as possible.

THE PRIVACY FORM NO ONE READS (AND SHOULD)

Every time we go to the doctor, the receptionist gives us forms to sign. Some of the forms ask extensive questions about our health background. Some forms tell us we must pay any bill that our insurance does not cover. Finally, some forms outline what the healthcare provider can and cannot do with our private health information. Wanting to be good patients, we rush to fill out and sign the required paperwork, rarely taking the time to truly read and understand our privacy rights. And if you ask the doctor's staff to explain, they often don't understand the rules themselves, nor do they have the time to explain your rights to you. But the reality is that the information contained in those privacy rights forms can have a tremendous impact on you.

WHAT IS HEALTHCARE PRIVACY?

What should you, as a patient, know about your healthcare privacy? Are doctors required to keep our health information private? Can they share our information without our permission? What information is protected? What are our rights as a parent to our child's health information? What happens when our healthcare privacy is compromised? This guide will answer these questions and more.

We must start with some basic information. First, what is **protected healthcare information** (PHI)? In the legal world, protected healthcare information is any written, spoken, or electronic information about your healthcare that also identifies you as the patient. PHI does not need to include your name. PHI can be any health information that also includes something that might lead to identifying you, such as your social security number, your address, your birthday, etc. Only under some limited circumstances may a healthcare provider give your PHI to someone without asking your permission. On the other hand, the healthcare provider can share information regarding your medical history if they take off anything that might identify you. This is known as de-identifying. Your name, social security number, address, date of birth, etc. must all be removed.

LAWS PROTECTING HEALTHCARE INFORMATION

In the United States, the formal protection of health information began in 1996 when the federal government passed the **Health Insurance Portability and Accountability Act (HIPAA)**. HIPAA requires any individual or group handling healthcare information (e.g. a doctor, hospital, or insurance company) to get written permission from a patient to disclose his or her healthcare information. Exceptions to this requirement include providing information to another treating physician, the patient's insurance company, or, in some limited circumstances, to law enforcement or the courts. When your healthcare provider asks you to sign a form granting them the right to give your health information to someone, it is important to read it and understand what rights you're giving up.

The HIPAA law was expanded in 2013 with the **Health Information Technology for Economic and Clinical Health Act (HITECH)**. The HITECH Act covers electronic health information and also expands the protections given to patients. Under the HITECH Act, if a healthcare provider hires a third party to help them with their patient information, the third party is also required to keep the patient's health information private. Third parties are generally companies that regularly help healthcare providers with their daily administrative tasks. The vendor maintaining the healthcare provider's electronic medical record or doing the billing has access to all the same information that the healthcare provider has to the patient's information, and under law should protect that information in the same way. As more people are accessing your health information, privacy is becoming more and more important.

So, what are the 10 things you need to know about your healthcare privacy?

1.

YOU OWN YOUR
MEDICAL RECORDS

This seems like a simple statement, but many people are confused about who owns their health information. Doctors, hospitals, and even patients sometimes make the mistake that since the medical professionals created the health record, they own it. This is simply not true. With very few exceptions, you own your health information and can review it at any time.

Your Records Aren't an Open Book

Imagine that you've seen the same primary doctor for twenty years who has helped you through not only colds and flu, but also through childbirth and post-partum depression, which she treated with medication over a decade ago. Now you need a knee replacement. Should your primary care doctor share all of your medical record with your new surgeon, including your treatment for depression? No. It is only appropriate for the primary care doctor to send the part of your health record that is relevant to the knee surgery, not the whole record. It is your choice to share with your new surgeon any additional information.

Likewise, if your doctor's office is using an outside billing company to bill insurance claims, the billing company must only be allowed to access the portions of the patient's record that are required to charge the visit to the insurance company. The billing company should not see anything unrelated to the claim being charged, such as previous treatment or identifying information, like a social security number, that is not relevant to the insurance company. The purpose of these restrictions is to keep as few people as possible from reviewing your health information. Limiting access to your records is the best way to limit breaches of your privacy.

You Control Who in Your Family Sees Your Records

Because you own your healthcare information, you are in charge of how it is shared with your family and loved ones. For example, if you prefer that your healthcare provider not use your home phone, but only call you on your cell phone, you can designate this choice. Or, for instance, if you have four adult children and you only want your healthcare provider to communicate with one of them, you also can designate this choice.

Making these choices known may be particularly important if you experience a life change such as a separation or divorce, or if you become a victim of domestic abuse.

Your Medical Records May Contain Mistakes

While healthcare providers work very hard to make sure your record is correct (no one wants a malpractice lawsuit), at times the wrong information can be included by mistake. This can occur, for example, when two patients have similar names. Or, laboratory results may have been excluded from your medical record. Since healthcare providers are taking care of many patients every day, mistakes can happen. Errors such as these can cause you to undergo unnecessary tests, receive the wrong care, or be denied life insurance or other benefits.

Ask to See Your Medical Records

You have the right to ask any healthcare provider for full access to your records at any time. That provider must also give you that access for free, but they can charge a reasonable fee for creating a copy of the record for you.

First, ask the office whether an authorization must be filled out. You are entitled to your own records, to those of your minor child (if your parental rights have not been revoked), and to those of any person for whom you are the legal guardian. If you want the medical records for an adult for whom you are not a legal guardian, you will need to have him or her sign an authorization allowing you to obtain their records. For a minor child, the guardian of that child must provide you with that permission in writing.

Ask How Long Your Doctor Will Keep Your Records

Normally, healthcare providers are required to keep a copy of your healthcare information for at least six years. States differ on the rules about the length of time for maintaining health information, but they will regularly be kept for six years or more. Some of the records may be electronic and some of the records may be paper. No matter what form the records are kept, a complete copy must be provided to you. Also, if you prefer to receive a copy of the records in electronic form, the doctor must provide it to you in that form.

Everything Takes Time

Of course, you cannot simply walk into your healthcare provider and demand to see your record immediately. You must give them a reasonable amount of time to make a copy or provide an opportunity to read it. Generally, healthcare providers have 30 days to give you a copy of the records after request them. Also, you should put your request in writing. If you need to get a copy of the record for an urgent purpose, you should state that in your written request and the healthcare provider should comply.

ASK AND YOU "SHOULD" RECEIVE

It is important to know that your medical file at one doctor's office may include your records from another doctor and that you are entitled to see those records as well.

This happens quite often. For example, when you see a new doctor for the first time, he or she may request the records from your previous doctor. This allows the new doctor to provide consistency in care and fully understand what care was provided previously. When a patient requests a copy of his or her record, doctors' offices are sometimes unsure if the patient is entitled to all of the records in the doctor's possession, even those which were provided by another doctor. It is important for you to know that anything in the doctor's record is yours.

THE "SQUEAKY WHEEL GETS THE GREASE"

If you have a hard time getting a copy of the record, ask who is in charge of the medical records. If you ask the receptionist at the office or hospital front desk for your record, your request might get lost with all the other work he or she has. On the other hand, many large doctors' offices have a privacy officer who can assist with your request. At a hospital or large facility, asking the medical records department for your file is usually a better and faster process for providing the records. Each state has different laws on how long the process can take, but all healthcare providers are required to produce the patient's medical records when asked.

REQUEST APPROPRIATE CHANGES

Because you own the information, you also have the right to request that the health record be amended or modified if you feel that a mistake has been made. Once the healthcare provider is alerted to the error, a correction or amendment is normally made in the health record in order to fix the mistake. This is one of the reasons why it is important to regularly review your records and the bills you receive to determine if there might be a problem.

However, being able to request an amendment or modification does not mean that if you simply disagree with the doctor, he or she is required to change your health record.

Similarly, some patients want their health record amended for insurance billing purposes. For example, your insurance plan may pay for a test to diagnose a problem. However, it will not pay if the test is a part of an annual screening. If your physician orders the test as a part of your annual physical, his or her office cannot, by law, change that fact in your record in order to have your insurance company pay for the test. A change or amendment can only be made if a genuine mistake has been in the health record.

DESIGNATE WHO IN YOUR FAMILY SEES YOUR RECORDS

When first visiting a healthcare provider make sure you let them know in writing who is allowed to view your medical records. Also, if you experience a life change such as a separation or divorce, make sure you update your information to exclude your estranged or former spouse if necessary. This is especially important if you are experiencing any kind of domestic abuse. Your healthcare provider is there to help you, and keeping your health information private is part of their job. If these issues are important to you, you should ask your healthcare provider how you make these designations.

KNOW WHEN YOU CAN'T SEE YOUR FILE

There are some limited exceptions when you might not be able to obtain your own health records. This normally involves mental health records. Certain mental health records will not be provided to the patient if the healthcare provider believes that the records will endanger the patient. It is not enough that the healthcare provider believes that patient will be upset when reviewing the health records. He or she must have a well-founded belief that viewing the record will cause the patient to harm himself or others. In less extreme situations, if you are denied access to your records, you should ask "why?"

THE BOTTOM LINE...

- Know that YOU own your healthcare records.

- Ask all of your healthcare providers to see your full medical record on a yearly basis.

- Ask to speak to the medical records department or privacy officer if you are asking for your records at a hospital or other large facility.

- Review your record for mistakes.

- Review your record to ensure that only the relevant parts of your medical history are being shared.

- Request corrections to mistakes in writing.

- Always let your healthcare providers know in writing who in your family can see your records.

- Always ask "why" when you are denied access to your records.

2.

How to Access (and Protect) the Medical Records of Your Child or Senior

As we have discussed, you own your medical record. But who owns the records of your loved ones? Let's start with your children.

SOLE CUSTODY DOESN'T MEAN SOLE RIGHT TO RECORDS

As long as your child remains a minor, both you and your child's other parent are entitled to a copy of his or her medical records. Sounds simple enough, but confusion can abound, particularly during and after custody battles.

On the most basic level, if your last name is different than the last name of your child, you may need to show proof that you are the parent when you request information about your child's care or medical records. Having your child's birth certificate handy during your first trip to the doctor's office, or when you ask for information, should be enough to clarify any questions.

What if the parents are divorced and one parent is awarded "sole custody" by the court? Many parents believe that if they have "sole custody," the non-custodial parent cannot see the child's medical records. This is simply not true. Unless the court has formally terminated the parental rights of the non-custodial parent, he or she is still entitled to their child's records. Likewise, what if only one parent is paying all the medical bills? Can the non-paying parent still have access to the records? The answer is "yes."

Issues around the status of a child's custody and the nature of the relationship between parents can often be confusing for healthcare workers so you might need to clarify if you are being wrongly denied access to your child's healthcare information, or if your child's records have been requested by a parent whose rights have been legally terminated.

Obviously, if there is a concern that the child is being abused by a parent, the other parent may go to the court to limit access to the records by the suspected mother or father. A court order will, however, likely be required to restrict access.

CARING FOR SENIORS (AND THEIR MEDICAL RECORDS)

More and more people are caring for an elderly family member in addition to their own immediate family. However, caring for a senior does not always mean that you are the guardian of that senior. In the world of law, most seniors are considered "legally competent," but in reality they need extensive help in managing their healthcare as they grow older and frailer. How then, do you ensure that your loved one's medical records are handled correctly?

The most important action you can take as a caregiver is to make sure that your senior designates you in writing as someone to whom a doctor or facility can provide medical information. If you have this signed authorization you will be able to get the information you need to help coordinate their care when they no longer can or need help in doing so.

If your loved one is moving to a rehabilitation facility, an assisted living facility, or a nursing home, the facility will need a copy of his or her medical records. Generally, the easiest option is to have the new facility request a copy of all the records directly from the healthcare providers (only medical facilities will have the ability to get these records without your loved one's authorization), or you can have your loved one sign an authorization asking the medical records to be sent to the facility. However the best option may be to have your loved one fill out an authorization that allows the records to be provided to you for transport. In doing so you can see what information is being shared with the facility, and it gives you the opportunity to make a copy of the record for any other need you or your senior might have at a later time.

If your loved one is already living in the nursing home, assisted living facility, or rehabilitation facility, the facility will send forms with the resident when he or she goes to an outside healthcare professional. That outside healthcare professional will then fill out the form to communicate what happened at the visit and what changes the facility should make to the senior's care as a result. Often those forms are returned to the facility via the healthcare provider's office.

However, it may make sense to have your senior sign an authorization for you to pick up the record and deliver it to the facility. Again, you and your loved one can monitor what is being communicated and you can keep a record for future needs.

THE BOTTOM LINE...

- If your last name is different than your child's i80, take a copy of your child's birth certificate with you on your child's first visit to a medical professional.

- Keep your child's healthcare provider up to date on any changes in custody, but understand that, unless his or her rights are legally terminated, your child's other parent is entitled to your child's medical records.

- If the parental rights of your child's other parent are legally terminated, let your healthcare provider know immediately.

- If you suspect abuse by the other parent, you must obtain a court order to deny the suspected parent access to your child's medical record.

- In caring for seniors, ensure that your loved one gives you written permission to access their medical records.

- When possible, personally transport your loved one's medical records so you can see what is being recorded and keep copies for future needs.

3.

Your Healthcare Provider Must Give You a Notice of Privacy (and You Must Read It)

By law, every healthcare provider must give you a copy of a **Notice of Privacy Practices**, which outlines how they will manage your information. The Notice will also list your rights by law, much of which is detailed in HIPAA and the HITECH Act. And while it is written in so much legalese, you must read the Notice thoroughly and change it to meet your own expectations regarding your privacy. The good news is that most doctors' Notices are very similar, so once you understand one, you can skim the others for changes.

THIS IS YOUR PRIVACY CONTRACT WITH YOUR DOCTOR

By signing a form confirming that you have read the Notice of Privacy Practices, you are saying that you agree to all of what they say they will do (or not do) in it. If later you disagree with how the doctor or other healthcare provider handled your information, and it was covered under the Notice, you won't have much chance of making them change.

REQUEST A COPY AND READ IT

Most healthcare providers will give you a copy of their Notice of Privacy Practices, but some may only give you a document to sign that says you were offered a copy of the Notice of Privacy Practices (giving you that paper being the "offer"). If you weren't given an opportunity to actually read the Notice, ask for a copy. It should also be on the healthcare providers' website and hanging in the lobby. Before you sign any confirmation, read the Notice. In particular, pay attention to the sections outlined below.

REVIEW THE SECTION ON ACCESS

First, the Notice will inform you about who will have access to your health information. All of the healthcare providers' staff, any volunteers, or medical students assisting with your care as well as any third parties contracted with the healthcare provider will likely have access to your health information. As the patient, if you do not want all of these people to review your health information, you should cross out what you will not agree to. For example, if you know some of the volunteers in the office and would prefer they not have access to your health information, you should inform the practice of your request.

REVIEW THE SECTION ON NOTIFICATION

Another important topic of the Notice of Privacy details how the healthcare provider will inform you about an upcoming appointment or test. It will tell you whether the healthcare provider will leave a message on your answering machine or voice mail. If you do not want to have such reminders, you need to cross out this portion of the Notice of Privacy Practices before you sign it, initial the change, and inform the staff that you have made a change. The healthcare provider is then not allowed to leave messages for you regarding your condition or test results unless you have specifically provided them with written authorization to do so.

REVIEW THE SECTION ON HEALTH DIRECTORIES

The healthcare provider will also tell you in the Notice of Privacy whether you will be included in any **health directory**. Health directories are often used in same-day surgery or in a hospital setting so your family can easily check to see how you are. It may simply list whether your procedure is completed and your general condition such as fair or good. If you do not want to be included in a health directory, you need to inform the healthcare provider. Again, if this is listed in the Notice make sure you cross it out, initial it, and point out the change to the office staff.

REVIEW THE SECTION ON RESEARCH

The Notice will also inform you about whether your health information will be used for research purposes. For some types of research, the healthcare provider must ask your specific permission. But for general research, the healthcare provider may tell you that they will use your information by listing it in the Notice of Privacy Practices. If you do not want to have your information used for research purposes, you should cross this section out.

KNOW YOUR PRIVACY OFFICER

Most importantly, the Notice of Privacy Practices will give the name of healthcare provider's Privacy Officer and his or her contact information. If there is a question or a problem with the confidentiality of your healthcare information, this is the person to contact.

THE BOTTOM LINE...

- Treat your doctor's Notice of Privacy Practices like a contract.

- If the healthcare provider doesn't provide you with a Notice, ask for a copy.

- Read it!

- Review key sections of the notice and amend them to meet your expectations.

- Make a note of who the healthcare provider's Privacy Officer is. Contact this person with any questions or problems.

4.

BE SMART WHEN COMMUNICATING WITH YOUR DOCTOR OVER THE WEB

It's very difficult to communicate with most doctors unless you make an appointment, take time to go to the office, pay a fee, and wait. We all have experienced calling the physician's office to ask a simple question only to end up on hold or never getting a promised return phone call. It's also normal after a short visit with the doctor to have a quick question you forgot to ask or to have something come up after the visit.

So, it's natural in this age of technology to think that a sending an email or text to your doctor is the perfect solution to the question. Instead it could leave you with far more problems.

MOST EMAILS AND TEXTS AREN'T SECURE

You need to remember that nothing is secure or private in emails or texts sent from cell phones or most email accounts (that includes both online accounts like Gmail or Yahoo! Mail AND your business or personal Outlook accounts). There is no guarantee that your email won't be sent mistakenly to someone else or that it will only be read by the medical professional to whom you sent it. Nor are you guaranteed that the response will be protected or private. Imagine the response to your question about a sensitive medical test going instead to another patient because your doctor accidentally copied a line from your file to the wrong email.

YOU MAY BE SIGNING AWAY YOUR PRIVACY RIGHTS

Be aware that if you send an email from your unsecure account to your doctor and ask for a response back to that account, you are waiving your privacy rights. Indeed, most doctors' offices will not allow this type of communication because they fear that it would violate HIPAA.

THE DOCTOR CAN'T SEE YOU NOW

A good doctor relies on his or her visual observations and the questions he or she asks of a patient before diagnosing a problem, giving advice, or writing a prescription. Because the doctor knows you will trust and rely on his or her answer, being right is crucial. Unlike an office visit, email and texts are forms of communication that limit the ability of the doctor to make the observations so critical to correctly addressing the needs of a patient.

This is why many healthcare providers will refuse to communicate with their patients via email or text regardless of whether the information is encrypted. The possibility of malpractice is too high.

SKIP THE EMAIL AND USE THE PATIENT PORTAL

As technology is expanding throughout healthcare, many healthcare professionals are starting to use a "patient portal" to communicate health information to their patients. The patient portal allows patients secure, 24/7 access to medical and billing information. The patient portal allows patients quick access to their medical information so they are better informed about their healthcare records.

As more healthcare providers use patient portals, you will be able to view recent doctor's visits, discharge summaries, medications, allergies, and lab results. You should also be able to make appointments, ask for prescription refills, check benefits, make payments, download necessary forms, and view educational materials.

You should check with your healthcare provider to find out if they have a patient portal or are developing one. If your doctor does have a patient portal, you can be confident that the information being passed across it is secure.

If You or Your Doctor Must Email or Text, Use Encryption

A simple way to protect your health information and also get a quick answer is to use **encryption** to send any email or text that might contain private health information. Encryption, very simply, is a key that you provide to your doctor that allows only the doctor to open the email and respond. If the email ends up going to someone else by mistake, it is unreadable without the key and so your privacy cannot be breached.

Many healthcare providers are now using encryption to communicate between doctors, hospitals, assisted living facilities, and other medical groups. The encryption keeps your information safe.

If your healthcare provider asks for your email, you should ask what information will be sent to you via email. If the information is private, you should ask whether the information will be sent in an encrypted format.

THE BOTTOM LINE...

- Do NOT email your doctor from an unsecured email account (e.g. Gmail, Yahoo! mail, Outlook).

- Ask your healthcare professional if his or her office has a patient portal. If so, use the portal for all online communication. If not, encourage him or her to invest in one.

- If you must email your doctor, encrypt your email.

- If your healthcare professional (or his or her office) wants to use email, ASK if he or she is using encryption. If not, say no thanks (and find another provider!).

5.

DOES YOUR HEALTHCARE PROVIDER USE AN ELECTRONIC HEALTH RECORD?

Many doctors and hospitals are moving from paper health records to **electronic health records** (EHRs). The terms "electronic medical record" and "electronic health record" are used interchangeably. An EHR is a digital record that includes your name, address, age, social security number, medical history, immunizations, allergies, medications, laboratory results, radiology imaging, personal information, and billing information. More and more healthcare providers are using EHRs to record patient visits. If you see your doctor using a laptop or computer to record your information, the doctor is most likely using an EHR.

Your EHR Can Be a Powerful Tool

Compared to paper records, EHRs can be a powerful tool in managing your healthcare. For example, EHRs can eliminate problems with reading the doctor's writing, a common complaint with paper records. With the EHR, everything is easy to read. Also, the EHR prompts the doctor to completely enter information about you during your visit, rather than at the end of the day when he or she is relying on memory. The consistency of the documentation in the EHR also allows other doctors in the practice to easily understand what happened at your last visit if they were not the one to see you. This is especially important when your healthcare provider is part of a large office or hospital.

Another advantage to the EHR is that all your medical records are stored in the same place. This is particularly helpful when your healthcare provider is trying to review your history. There is no need to chase down all of your records if your healthcare provider has scanned them into the EHR.

EHRs Can Be Difficult to Share with Patients

While EHRs have many advantages over paper records, there are potential issues to keep in mind. A basic concern involves whether or not your healthcare provider can easily provide you with a printed or electronic copy of your EHR at your request, which they are required by law to do. This seems like a simple question, but many EHR software providers have difficulty supporting the export of a patient's full record into a printable or downloadable file. Administrative staff at your healthcare provider will also have different skill levels when it comes to using EHR software.

How Secure Is Your EHR?

Let's face it. Breaches of electronic data happen every day. Whether you are Target or the Pentagon, breaches are going to happen. As EHRs become more common in healthcare, we benefit from the efficiencies the EHR creates, but we also have to be aware that our health information is at risk. Healthcare providers have computers or laptops stolen. Criminally-minded staff inappropriately access someone's health information for identity theft. Someone hacks into healthcare information because it's not properly secured.

The government requires healthcare providers to have security policies and procedures in place to ensure that they are taking all reasonable and necessary precautions to protect their patients' health information. Also, HIPAA requires healthcare providers to take higher security measures for EHRs than for paper records. For example, they are required to have the proper hardware and software protections for the information. Your healthcare provider must also have an audit trail of who has accessed your EHR. If your healthcare information is compromised, an audit trail allows the provider to easily see who viewed your records and when.

It is also important to remember that breaches of your health information can be from within the healthcare provider's office or external to the office, and that the breach can be intentional or unintentional. Also remember that anyone reviewing your medical record must have a legitimate, healthcare-related reason to be looking at your record and must have your authorization.

ASK FOR A COPY

Request a copy of your EHR after you have seen the provider a few times. This will give you a good indication of what your healthcare provider can download from the system when you request a copy of your record in the future.

OBSERVE HOW YOUR DOCTOR'S OFFICE TREATS YOUR DATA

As a patient, it is important to be aware of what the healthcare provider is doing to protect your information. Is the healthcare provider using encryption to protect against unauthorized access to the health record? Is the computer screen open and readable by anyone entering the office? Are the healthcare providers using passwords before they can enter data? Are they logging in and out when different providers enter data? Every healthcare provider using an EHR has an obligation to take these steps to protect your health information.

DON'T ASK FOR INAPPROPRIATE INFORMATION

It is inappropriate for a healthcare worker to access a patient's EHR to look up information for someone such as a friend or relative if that individual is not involved in the care of the patient. Something as simple as looking in your medical record to obtain your address or phone number to contact you about something unrelated to your care is a breach. You should never ask a friend or relative who works for a hospital or healthcare facility to help you gain unofficial access to your health records or those of someone else. You are asking them to break the law.

THE BOTTOM LINE...

- Ask if your doctor uses Electronic Health Records (EHRs).

- If so, ask for a copy of yours.

- Find out what safeguards your doctor's office has around their EHRs.

- Observe how your doctor's office treats your EHR.

- NEVER ask for information from an EHR that you are not entitled to.

- NEVER accept information from an EHR that you are not entitled to.

6.

ASK IF YOUR PROVIDER USES A HEALTH INFORMATION EXCHANGE

Relatively new to the scene, **Health Information Exchanges (HIEs)** are systems that allow your healthcare information to be immediately accessed and updated by all of your caregivers. HIEs are meant to replace old paper-based communication methods and to allow the computer systems of large health systems to talk to each other. If put into operation properly, HIEs will potentially revolutionize how health information is shared.

When your healthcare provider joins an HIE, he or she agrees to allow their electronic health records to be easily read by other healthcare providers under the rules outlined in HIPAA and the HITECH Act. Everyone who is a member of the HIE can access other providers' records to quickly determine what medications the patient is taking, what allergies or health conditions he or she has, and other important information.

HEALTH RECORDS AREN'T IMMEDIATELY AVAILABLE IN AN EMERGENCY

Right now, when you have a sudden illness you may be transported by an ambulance, seen in an emergency room, admitted to the hospital, and cared for by numerous healthcare providers who work for different companies. All of these healthcare providers will either create a new medical record for you or access their own record of your care in their own system if one exists. And without an HIE, the chances of all those records being quickly available in an emergency are slim. The paramedics would not know exactly what medications you were taking prior to your illness. The emergency room doctor could not immediately see what medications were administered during the ambulance transport, nor could she have easy access to your cardiologist's records or your internist records.

LACK OF INFORMATION CAN LEAD TO DELAYS AND POOR CARE

If your regular doctor is not **credentialed** to practice at the hospital where you were taken, you will likely be assigned a new, unfamiliar doctor who will have to wait to receive your records from your primary care physician and, sometimes, make decisions without them. You can face the same issue when discharged to a rehabilitation facility or long-term care facility with its own medical record system outside of the hospital. Moreover, if you are admitted to receive care at one of these facilities on the weekend, you will likely not be able to obtain your health records from your doctor until their office opens on Monday. All of these missing pieces of your health information can lead to mistakes or delays in your care.

ENCOURAGE YOUR DOCTOR TO PARTICIPATE IN AN *HIE*

Currently most HIEs are in the development stage or can only share basic information such as prescription information. However, this is rapidly changing as more and more healthcare providers are utilizing electronic health records. If you are interested in making sure that your health information can be transferred quickly and securely between all your healthcare providers, ask if they participate in a HIE. If not encourage them to do so.

KNOW YOUR *HIE*

If your healthcare provider does participate in an HIE, ask which one it is. Depending on where you live, there may be many HIEs available, such as in a large urban area. If your doctor is affiliated with a specific health system, they will likely use the same HIE that the health system is using. This is important to remember when you have a choice of where to go for urgent care or emergency care.

Staying within one HIE will greatly assist you in getting all your medical records to the new provider in a secure manner.

THE BOTTOM LINE...

- Understand how a Health Information Exchang (HIE) works.

- Ask your healthcare providers participate in an HIE.

- Know the name of your healthcare providers' HIE.

- When possible, choose hospitals and urgent care facilities within that HIE.

7.

KEEP YOUR OWN RECORD OF ALL IMPORTANT HEALTH INFORMATION

While advances in information technology are happening every day in healthcare, the industry still has a long way to go. Many healthcare providers still use paper medical records, and if they do use electronic medical records, their software likely won't talk to the software being used by other healthcare professionals, unless they are participating in an HIE. Because of these challenges, many healthcare providers will place the burden of obtaining health records on the patient. Therefore, be prepared to act as the keeper of your own medical record and those of your loved ones.

MAKE A MEDICAL LIFE LIST, KEEP CHECKING IT

When you are sick or have a family member who needs immediate medical attention, you rarely have the time or the resources to gather health information. Therefore, it is important that, before an emergency happens, you create a record of all important health information for you and your loved ones that you can easily refer to, something we call a Medical Life List.

The list should include your personal information such as name, address, social security information, driver's license number, employer, and insurance provider (including your group number). Next, the list should detail all of your healthcare providers' information such as their names, addresses, specialties, and hospital affiliation.

Next, you should include any information about major health events, including any hospitalizations and changes in insurance. A Medical Life List should also detail any medications being taken and allergies you or your loved one has. Also, for children, you should keep track of illnesses, vaccinations and days of missed school.

Remember to update your Medical Life List when you or your loved one adds or changes a doctor or medication as well as the date for when the change happened. Always keep the list in a secure format and shred any old copies. If you are comfortable with computers and can keep a digitally encrypted copy of the list, keep only an electronic copy. However, if you prefer to keep a paper copy, do so. You should also have the list readily available in case of an emergency. Finally, your loved ones should know where the list is and have access to it if they need to assist with your healthcare.

In addition to the list, you should keep copies of important medical records, tests, and laboratory results.

AVOID UNNECESSARY TESTS AND PROCEDURES

Having copies of your prior tests and procedures will help you avoid unnecessary tests. We've all heard stories about healthcare providers who ordered too many tests or unnecessary procedures simply because they did not have an accurate picture of a patient's treatment history. While repeating a test may sometimes be necessary, you can short-circuit unneeded procedures (and the bills for them) by simply keeping copies of the tests and results with you.

MANY CAREGIVERS, MANY POTENTIAL PROBLEMS

When care is spread across several healthcare providers, it becomes even more crucial for patients or their loved ones to accurately record and communicate their medical information to everyone involved.

This is especially important if you are caring for an elderly parent or spouse. As we age, our healthcare needs tend to get more complicated, and it can be difficult for the senior patient to track his or her complex healthcare information. In general, seniors receive most of their healthcare at the end of their lives. As an elderly patient has more chronic problems as they age, their healthcare will become more involved, and the room for potential errors grows. It is essential for the healthcare provider to get a current Medical Life List of medications and updated health information each time the elderly patient receives care, since it likely will have changed since their last visit. As more and more families are taking care of an elderly parent or spouse, keeping up-to-date medical information that is secure and private is essential.

KEEP A CALENDAR TO KEEP IT SIMPLE

Many people must keep track of a healthcare list for loved ones who live independently but aren't able or willing to capture changes to their treatment. For example, your elderly father may visit the doctor alone, but will forget to update his list with new prescriptions or test results. A simple way to ask your loved ones to keep track of their important healthcare changes is to give them a special calendar, which shows all healthcare appointments. He or she can then use the calendar to write down what happened at the appointment. You can then regularly check the calendar to update the healthcare list.

DON'T LEAVE HOME WITHOUT IT

If you are going to a new doctor or something in your health has changed, simply take your Medical Life List with you to the office. The doctor will likely put a copy of the list in your medical chart, or you can use your list to accurately fill out the required forms at the doctor.

Also don't assume that every healthcare provider knows your medical history by heart. If you feel your doctor, physician's assistant, or other health professional has forgotten something or has misinterpreted your medical information or that of your loved one, use your Medical Life List to ensure that you and your healthcare worker have a common understanding of your medical record.

IDENTIFY "OWNERS" OF MEDICATIONS

Make sure your list details which healthcare provider will be in charge of which medications. This is particularly crucial in caring for elderly patients. The prescribing of Lasix, a common medication used to remove excess fluid in the elderly, is a simple example of how important ownership can be. Internists often adjust the Lasix dosage as do cardiologists and nephrologists, but if each doctor continues to adjust the Lasix dosage with no coordination between them, there will likely be a mistake in how much Lasix the patient receives, leading to serious complications. By simply identifying with the doctors' input who should be the only one to adjust the Lasix dosage, you can avoid a major problem. This is true of many different medications.

PERSONAL HEALTH RECORDS (PROCEED WITH CAUTION)

Many technologies are being developed to help patients capture and manage their healthcare information. These new technologies include the **personal health record**. Offered by online companies (e.g. WebMD) and healthcare providers alike, personal health records can take on many forms, but have a common concept: providing the patient with one electronic location to keep all copies of your health records. This location may be on an external device (e.g. a flash drive), on a company's own internal servers, or in "the cloud."

It is important to note that many of the companies offering personal health records are not classified by the government as healthcare providers. As a result, their storage of your healthcare information will be governed by Federal Trade Commission's (FTC) health information rules, not HIPAA. This is a significant distinction since far more protections exist under the HIPAA/HITECH law than under the FTC. Healthcare companies also know severe penalties apply to violations of HIPAA, an extra motivation to make every effort to protect your personal information.

PERSONAL HEALTH RECORD "PROS"

A personal health record will likely be a great resource in the future. When all your health information is easily accessible to you, it is often easier to understand and ask questions. It provides an easy way for a new healthcare provider or caregiver to become knowledgeable about your healthcare needs. It also allows you to gain access to your medical information when you are traveling and can be a useful tool when your doctor's office is closed.

PERSONAL HEALTH RECORD "CONS"

A personal health record, however, is only as good as the company providing the service. You should make sure that any company you choose to maintain your healthcare information is stable and likely to be in business for a long time. If you rely on a start-up company to maintain your health records and that company closes, you will likely lose access to your electronic file and may need to gather your information all over again.

Healthcare providers also have concerns about new companies gathering health records for a patient. Since these products are in the development phase, your healthcare provider may still want to gather your records independently so they can be certain the records are authentic. Also a personal health record provides yet another location for a privacy breach, so make sure the company you're using has a high level of security around your sensitive data.

If you are considering using a personal health record company, you should weigh the risks and the benefits prior to providing that company with access to your healthcare information. Also, a personal healthcare record should not be a substitute for a list of healthcare providers, medications, and other important health information you keep at your fingertips. In an emergency, you may not be able to access your personal health record, so your Medical Life List is always a great resource for you and your family.

THE BOTTOM LINE...

- Make and keep updated a Medical Life List of your important health information.

- Always take that list with you to the doctor's office and other healthcare visits.

- Keep copies of your medical procedures and tests results to avoid unnecessary treatment.

- Make sure all your healthcare providers know which professional manages each medication taken by you or your loved one.

- Have your loved one keep a calendar with their medical appointments.

- Carefully evaluate any service providing personal health records, including their company health, security practices, and if they are governed by HIPAA laws.

8.

DESIGNATE WHO IN YOUR LIFE HAS ACCESS TO YOUR HEALTH INFORMATION

If you cannot make a decision for yourself, a medical professional is allowed to share your health information with family members, partner, or close friend so they can make that decision on your behalf. However, it's up to the healthcare professional to choose that person if you haven't made your preference officially known. If you do have a preference, then you must let your doctor know in writing. The only exception occurs when the patient is a minor. When a doctor is caring for a minor, both parents are entitled to the health information, even if one or the other states otherwise.

Your Wishes May Not Be Honored

In most circumstances, healthcare professionals don't know the exact nature of your relationship with family, and can only use their own judgment to determine who should speak or act on your behalf. The doctor may not know you are estranged from your spouse or have adult children you don't want involved in your healthcare. Also, in circumstances where you cannot make decisions about your care, the doctor may speak to someone who has no idea what your actual wishes are, and, as a result, will not honor them.

The Person You Want May Not Be a Family Member

What if you have a significant person in your life you want to act your behalf but is not a relative? If you haven't outlined this in writing, you may have difficulty getting your health information to him or her, or in having that person's voice heard above those of relatives when you cannot speak for yourself. Also, if you rely on a neighbor or a close friend to help you get to your appointments or care for you when you are ill, you will need to give your healthcare provider an authorization to release your information to him or her. Otherwise that friend will be unable to help you when you need them the most.

COMMUNICATE YOUR CHOICE IN WRITING

Whomever you are going to select to have access to your health-care information, the choice should be in writing. Without a designation in writing, your healthcare provider will be limited as to who they can talk to. In an emergency or when battling a life-threatening illness, you do not want your healthcare providers to be unsure about your wishes. Also, if you fail to give written directions, it is easier for your healthcare provider to simply refuse to share any information, rather than risk violating your confidentiality and legal rights.

It is always difficult to choose between many people or even pick one person to have access to your medical records. Your healthcare is private and important so many people avoid the choice. If you have several adult children, do you want all of them to have access to your records? You might consider selecting one or two of them who live close by and are likely to be with you if you are sick or cannot care for yourself.

DESIGNATE A PATIENT ADVOCATE

You may also want to designate a **patient advocate**. Although the terminology can vary from state to state, a patient advocate is the one person whom the doctor can communicate with in the event that you cannot participate in your own healthcare decisions. The patient advocate will also know your wishes regarding treatment and end-of-life choices in the case of terminal illness or a serious accident.

It is also helpful for you to have an "**advanced directive**." Again, the terminology can vary state to state, but generally an advance directive is a document signed by you that clearly outlines your wishes for life-saving measures and healthcare options that may prolong your life. Many people feel differently about end-of-life issues. It is important to discuss these issues with your patient advocate and others in your life in advance of a healthcare crisis, no matter how difficult the conversation. You should also make sure to keep these documents in a secure location so this information is readily available in case of an emergency.

THE BOTTOM LINE...

- Determine who in your life should have access to your healthcare information (can be more than one person).

- Speak to that person or persons.

- Inform your healthcare professionals about your choice in writing.

- Designate a patient advocate (one person).

- Speak to that person.

- Inform your healthcare professionals about your choice in writing.

- Consider having an advanced directive.

9.

What to Do If Your Private Information Is Compromised

As we've seen, good healthcare providers take every necessary precaution to protect your data, but no system is perfect, and mistakes—or in some cases crimes—can occur.

Stories of breaches in healthcare information fill new sites every day. For example, in July 2013, Chicago's largest physician group (more than 1,000 doctors) had four computers stolen, placing at risk the private data of over four million patients, including their names and Social Security numbers. In the same month one of the nation's largest insurance companies exposed the protected health information of over 600,000 patients on the Internet. Because the company had no safeguards verifying who accessed the information, the government fined them $1.7 million. Two months later, a California medical center had a patient care laptop stolen from an employee's car. The laptop contained the unencrypted health information of over 3,500 patients.

As you can see, patient health information breaches are not isolated occurrences. Therefore, you need to review any notices you receive from your healthcare providers about any breach of your healthcare information and determine what steps you need to take. You must also take the steps to monitor your healthcare information.

HEALTHCARE PROVIDERS *MUST* NOTIFY YOU IF A BREACH OCCURS

If a data breach of your healthcare information occurs, the healthcare provider must notify you within 60 days or less of its discovery. HIPAA and the HITECH Act have placed many specific obligations on healthcare providers regarding breach notifications to patients. These rules are intended to provide the patients with a quick, complete notice so they can take action to minimize the effects of the breach. For example, if your social security number and other important information are compromised, you can quickly review your credit to determine if you have become a victim of identity theft. The requirement to notify is also intended to encourage healthcare providers to secure their patients' health data as much as possible. No sane healthcare professional wants to send a breach notification if it can be avoided.

When a healthcare provider discovers a potential breach, they are required to perform a risk assessment to determine whether there was indeed a breach, how the breach occurred, who was involved, and whether they should notify the patients. They are also required to take action to ensure the breach will not occur again.

IF IT'S BIG ENOUGH, THE MEDIA MUST BE INVOLVED

In September 2013, the HITECH Act, in response to evolving technology, revised the standard as to what sort of breach requires patient notification. If the health data involved in the breach was encrypted, then notification is unnecessary since the data cannot be read by anyone who does not have the encryption key.

In the case of unencrypted data, however, the HITECH Act took a different approach. Before, when a breach of any kind occurred, healthcare providers did not have to immediately assume the breach harmed patients. Therefore, they could evaluate the seriousness of the breach and, with guidance, decide whether or not to notify patients. After the HITECH Act, however, any compromise of unencrypted data now carries with it an immediate assumption of harm, making it almost certain that the healthcare provider must inform affected patients.

In addition to informing patients of the breach, a healthcare provider may have to alert the media if the breach involves over 500 patients. The healthcare provider must also inform the Secretary of Health and Human Services (HHS). Large breach notifications are available to the public to review on the HHS website. The public list of breach notifications will provide the name of the healthcare provider, when the breach occurred, how many individuals were impacted, and a summary of the breach. The database can also be searched to find a specific healthcare provider or a certain type of breach. To view HHS breach notifications go to: http://www.hhs.gov/ocr/privacy/hipaa/administrative/breachnotificationrule/breachtool.html

IF YOU DISCOVER THE BREACH, ALERT THE PRIVACY OFFICER

How will you know if your healthcare has been breached? People find out many different ways. For example, your employer asks to speak with you about your HIV status, which has become known in the workplace. Maybe you "google" your name and you see your health insurance information posted on a public website. Or your daughter's private health information becomes a topic of gossip at her high school.

If any suspected breach occurs, you want to immediately notify your healthcare provider. A healthcare provider who takes their patients' privacy seriously will want to know if a problem exists or a crime has occurred. If you do not have the name of the Privacy Officer (often listed on the Notice of Privacy), simply call the healthcare provider and ask for that person. Have as much information as possible about the suspected breach. Your healthcare provider is obligated to immediately investigate the breach, but without good evidence of the breach, it may be difficult to find the source.

IF YOUR HEALTHCARE PROVIDER ALERTS YOU, TAKE ACTION

When your healthcare provider discovers the breach, they will send you a letter, and, once you are notified, you should take immediate action. Your healthcare provider is required to give you a description of how the breach occurred, what you can do to protect yourself, and what the healthcare provider is doing to protect your health information going forward. If the breach involved access to your financial information, social security number, or credit card, you should ask your healthcare provider to pay for a credit monitoring service to guard against future identity theft.

FILE A COMPLAINT WITH THE GOVERNMENT IF APPROPRIATE

If you believe a breach of your healthcare information has occurred and your healthcare provider is unresponsive or hostile, you can file a complaint with U.S. Health and Human Services Office of Civil Rights. You can file the complaint in writing or electronically. The link for filing a complaint is: http://www.hhs.gov/ocr/privacy/hipaa/complaints/ You must file the complaint within 180 days of the breach occurring or when you discovered the breach.

Penalties for healthcare providers who compromise patient data are growing. The penalties are greater when the healthcare provider should have known HIPAA violations existed. Penalties range from $100 to $50,000 per violation if they did NOT know there was a violation. The penalties increase to $1,000 to $50,000 per violation if the provider should have reasonably known about the violation. The highest penalty of $50,000 per violation is accessed when the healthcare provider willfully neglected their HIPAA responsibilities and did nothing to correct the breach. These penalties can grow very quickly since most breaches involve many patients and the penalties can be accessed on each patient breach.

THE BOTTOM LINE...

- If you discover that your private health information has been compromised, alert your healthcare provider's Privacy Officer.

- If you are alerted to a breach, work with the Privacy Officer to determine the nature of the breach.

- If appropriate, check your credit immediately and work with your credit companies and local law enforcement to combat fraud and identity theft.

- If necessary, file a complaint with the U.S. Health and Human Services Office of Civil Rights.

10.

You Must Keep Your Healthcare Information Private

After reviewing the obligations of healthcare providers, we need to look at our own actions in order to protect our healthcare information.

You Are Your Own Best Friend (or Worst Enemy)

The first place to start when maintaining your health privacy is with you. You and your family have the most access to all your health information and you should be protecting it. You can't blame your healthcare provider for a breach if you cannot determine whether the breach actually came from the healthcare provider or rather you or your family.

Safe Places

First, you should not talk openly in public spaces about your family's healthcare. At a restaurant, in a lobby, or at work are not proper locations to discuss your sensitive health issues. If you want to keep your health information private, be cautious about where you are discussing it.

Additionally, you should maintain your healthcare information in a safe place. It should not be thrown into a pile on your desk at work or left in a public place. If you are throwing away a copy of a health test or a health insurance bill make sure to shred the information beforehand.

Keep Your Computer Protected

The same is true if you have health information stored on your computer. If the computer is being used by others, you should password protect any information that you do not want others to access. Never store health information on your employer's computer. All information you save to or email from your employer's computer is the property of your employer. If this information is private, you need to maintain it on a separate computer you own. If you are concerned about keeping your health information private, it must start with you.

Always follow good practices when selecting your password. Don't pick something anyone can guess. The easiest password to guess is "123456." If there is a password that everyone knows you use, do not use it for private health information. Additionally, you should not post your password anywhere in plain sight. People often put a sticky note on their computer so they have their passwords close at hand. This is not a good practice if you are trying to keep your healthcare or anything else private. Lastly, you should not share your password with anyone.

Post Nothing on Social Media You Don't Want the World to See

Remember there is nothing private about social media. If you have a Facebook, Twitter, or other social media account and you update your family and friends on your healthcare status via that account, know that is a public place where the information can be accessible by others. Additionally, everything posted on the internet will remain there forever. If the information is private, social media is not a place to communicate with others about your or your family's healthcare.

Choose Your Mobile Devices Wisely

Many mobile devices are now being offered to capture or monitor your health information. For example, some doctor's offices offer patients iPads or apps in order to keep track of blood pressure, weight, sugar levels, etc. If you choose to use a mobile device for any of your healthcare needs, you should make sure to research the device or program. If a healthcare provider does not offer the healthcare product, the healthcare laws will not bind the company that does. Be certain that the healthcare product is offered by a trusted company.

Make sure to read all the privacy notices and security before you enter any of your healthcare information. As discussed earlier, using encryption with the healthcare device will protect the information. Without encryption, the information is likely to be breached. It is always helpful if the device has an ability to wipe the information clean if your mobile device is stolen or lost. Taking the time to make sure the mobile product is secure before you enter your health information is well worth your time and energy.

BE A PARTNER TO YOUR DOCTOR'S OFFICE

An important gauge of determining if your healthcare provider takes your health privacy seriously is to simply observe their office. Are computers on with information easily viewed? Are there paper charts, test results, or other documents lying around the patient areas? Can you easily overhear conversations by the office staff on the phone with other patients about important private health matters? If the healthcare provider takes your privacy seriously, everyone working for them will behave accordingly. If you see or hear anything in your doctor's office that causes you concern, share that concern constructively with the Privacy Officer. Chances are he or she will be grateful to have an issue brought to their attention before it becomes a breach.

Conversely, it is important to know when healthcare providers are allowed to have conversations with their patients even if another person might overhear them. A simple example of this can be when a doctor visits his patient in a semi-private room in a hospital. The other patient in the room along with their family is likely to overhear what the doctor is saying. However, HIPAA provides for such exceptions because they are unavoidable. This is also true of calling your name in your doctor's waiting room. The doctor is also allowed to assume that if you have someone with you at the time of your doctor's visit that they may talk to you about your private health information in front of that person.

THE BOTTOM LINE...

- Do NOT discuss sensitive health issues in public.

- If you store health information on your computer or mobile device, use a strong password to protect it.

- Do NOT store health information on a work computer or laptop.

- Do NOT post sensitive health information on social media.

- Make sure any mobile device for monitoring your healthcare is secure and offered by a reputable company.

- Share any concerns you have regarding how a doctor's office protects patient information with the Privacy Officer.

CONCLUSION

As you can see, as healthcare continues to change, healthcare privacy remains a challenge. Everyone has a different level of comfort about what healthcare information they openly disclose and what information they prefer to keep private. People differ on what amount of privacy they are willing to give up for easier access to their health information. As healthcare technology develops, privacy concerns will continue to grow. You must take charge of your healthcare and be informed about the options available. The more you know the more you will feel in control of your healthcare information and needs.

TERMS TO KNOW

Advanced directive: A legal document signed by you that clearly outlines your wishes for life-saving measures and healthcare options that may prolong your life.

Credentialed: Term referring to a physician's ability to practice medicine at a given hospital. Administrators will regularly review a physician's training, practice history, and certifications among other factors to determine if he or she may practice at their hospital.

Electronic health record (EHR): A digital record that includes your name, address, age, social security number, medical history, immunizations, allergies, medications, laboratory results, radiology imaging, personal information, and billing information. May also be called a "electronic medical record."

Encryption: A method for protecting electronic data in which the sender provides a key to the recipient so only that recipient can view the data. Encryption can be used to send sensitive data to your doctor via email if needed.

Health directory: A source for patients' family and friends to receive updates on that patient while he or she is in receiving treatment at a hospital or other facility.

Health information exchange (HIE): System that allows your healthcare information to be immediately accessed and updated by all of your caregivers. An HIE is meant to replace old paper-based communication methods and to allow the computer systems of large health systems to talk to each other.

Health Insurance Portability and Accountability Act (HIPAA): U.S. federal law governing how the healthcare industry should maintain the privacy and security of individually identifiable health information.

Information Technology for Economic and Clinical Health Act ("HITECH"): Expansion of HIPAA that covers electronic health information and expands the privacy protections given to patients.

Notice of Privacy Practices: Legal document given to you by a healthcare provider that outlines how they will manage your private information. The Notice of Privacy Practices will also list your rights by law, much of which is detailed in HIPAA and the HITECH Act.

Patient advocate: The person legally designated by you as the one whom the doctor can communicate with in the event that you cannot participate in your own healthcare decisions. The patient advocate will also know your wishes regarding treatment and end-of-life choices in the case of terminal illness or a serious accident.

Personal health record: A product or service that provides patients with one electronic location to keep all copies of their health records.

Protected healthcare information (PHI): In the legal world, any written, spoken or electronic information about your healthcare that also identifies you as the patient. Identifying information can include your name, social security number, address, birthday, etc.

Third party: In the context of healthcare, companies that regularly help medical practices and other providers with their daily administrative tasks, such as billing or record management.

LORI-ANN'S ON YOUR SIDE

"When I need health care advice I can understand and follow, I call Lori-Ann. She knows her stuff!"
M. Diane Vogt, JD

"Lori-Ann is my "go-to" expert on healthcare law. She makes it understandable and easy to follow for our doctors and their patients, too."
Michele Nichols, The Physician Alliance

"Lori-Ann knows the healthcare system inside and out. Whenever we have questions about healthcare, Lori-Ann has the answers."
Mike Gerstenlauer, St. John-Macomb Hospital

"Whenever my family has a health care issue, Lori-Ann is my first call for the best advice."
Donna Curran

"Getting coverage for prescription drugs can be a big problem for patients. Lori-Ann knows the insider secrets to making it easy."
Coreen Buehrer

"Lori-Ann has also lived the difficult issues that families confront on a daily basis as they struggle with the bewildering maze of hospitals, multiple specialists and insurance companies as our family's tireless advocate for our father. No mother grizzly ever fought for her cubs with more passion than Lori-Ann looked out for our dad."
Stephen Rickard, J.D., MPA

ABOUT THE AUTHOR

Lori-Ann Rickard is one of the country's top healthcare lawyers. For over three decades, she has advised leading hospitals, doctors, laboratories, and other healthcare providers. Now she offers her expertise to patients and their families through the Easy Healthcare Series from HealthSpin.

Lori-Ann is also a single mom of two beautiful daughters. One of her daughters was very sick when she was born. Already caring for a toddler and managing a developing career, Lori-Ann used her professional experience to create quick, effective strategies to make the healthcare system work for her as she sought the best treatment possible for her sick baby. Later, Lori-Ann served as the primary caregiver and medical coordinator for her proud, independent parents when they became unable to care for themselves. Through their wellness challenges, her daughter's illness, and in helping friends over the past thirty years, Lori-Ann has used her unique position in the industry to create easy healthcare solutions that work for everyone around her. These solutions will work for you and your family, too.

Lori-Ann Rickard is a healthcare insider who knows what it means to be a patient and a caregiver. The Easy Healthcare Series brings you the benefit of Lori-Ann Rickard's expertise. Let her show you how you can Spin Your Healthcare Your Way.

More By Lori-Ann Rickard

Visit myhealthspin.com to download your free copy
of *Easy Healthcare: What You Need First!*
ALSO AVAILABLE FROM HEALTHSPIN:

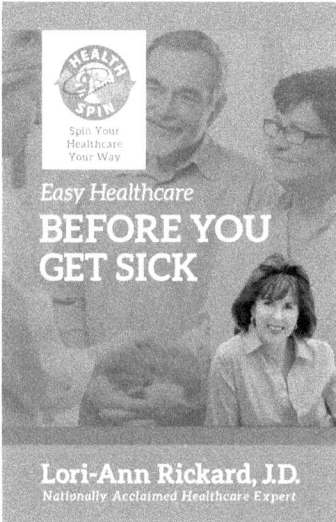

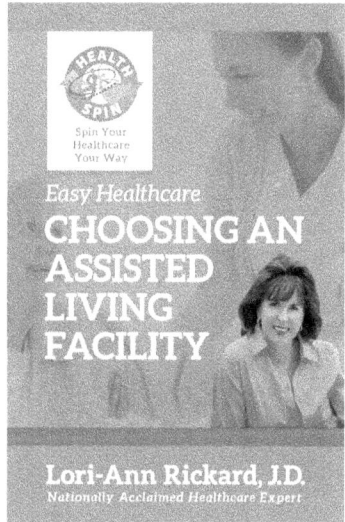

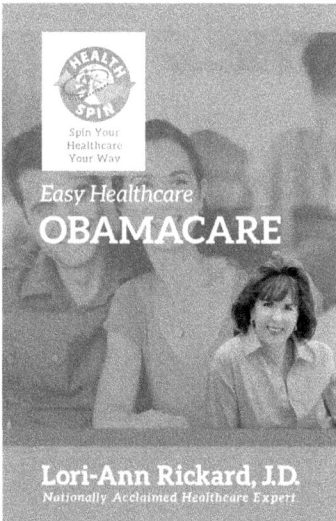

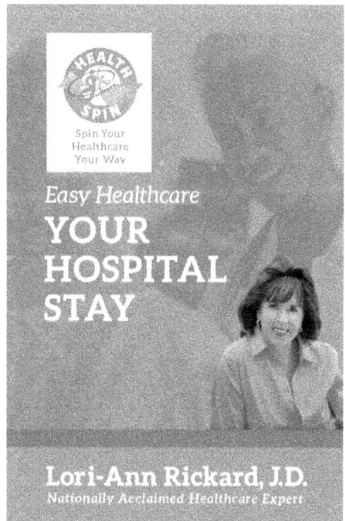

Easy Healthcare
BEFORE YOU GET SICK
Lori-Ann Rickard, J.D.
Nationally Acclaimed Healthcare Expert

Easy Healthcare
CHOOSING AN ASSISTED LIVING FACILITY
Lori-Ann Rickard, J.D.
Nationally Acclaimed Healthcare Expert

Easy Healthcare
OBAMACARE
Lori-Ann Rickard, J.D.
Nationally Acclaimed Healthcare Expert

Easy Healthcare
YOUR HOSPITAL STAY
Lori-Ann Rickard, J.D.
Nationally Acclaimed Healthcare Expert